Snowball, the white mouse

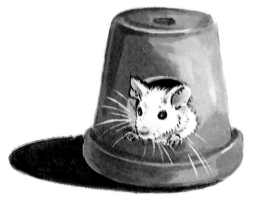

Story by Hugh Price   **Illustrations by Betty Greenhatch**

Snowball was a little white mouse.

He did not like the pet shop.

"I don't like kittens and puppies,"
he said.   "They **eat** mice."

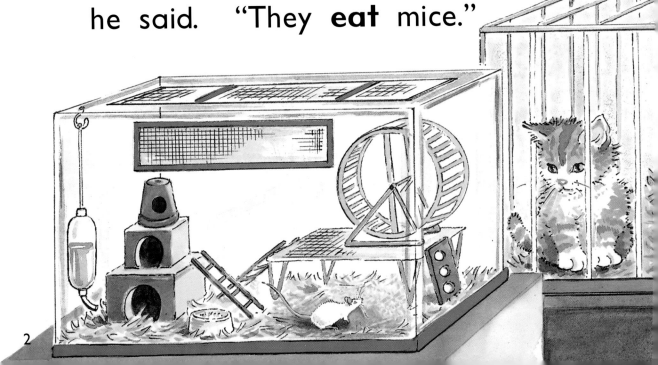

"I want someone to come
and buy me," he said.

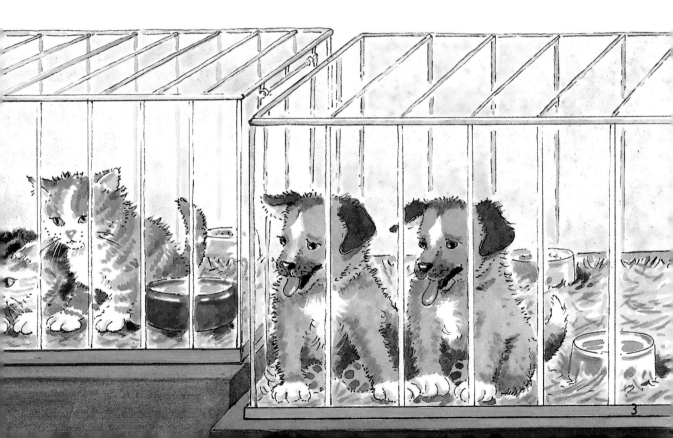

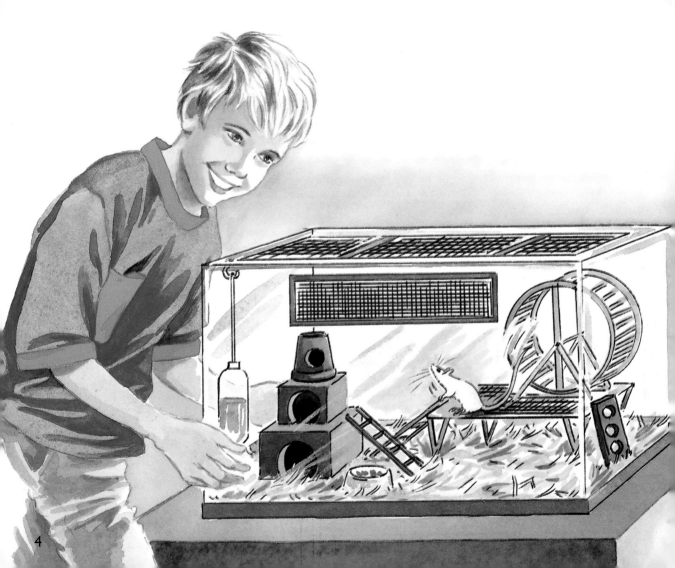

A boy came into the shop.

"I have a kitten at home,"

he said.

"If I buy a mouse,

I will have **two** pets."

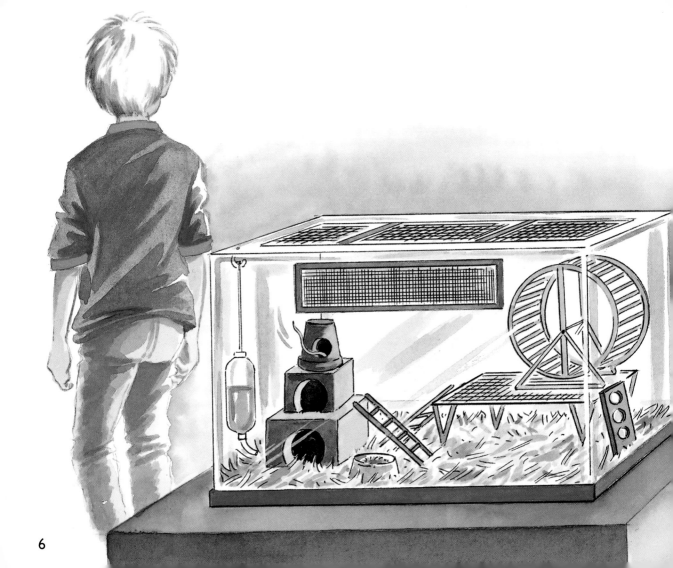

Snowball said, "Kittens eat mice!
I don't want that boy to buy me."

Snowball ran up the ladder
to his little room and hid inside.

The boy walked away.

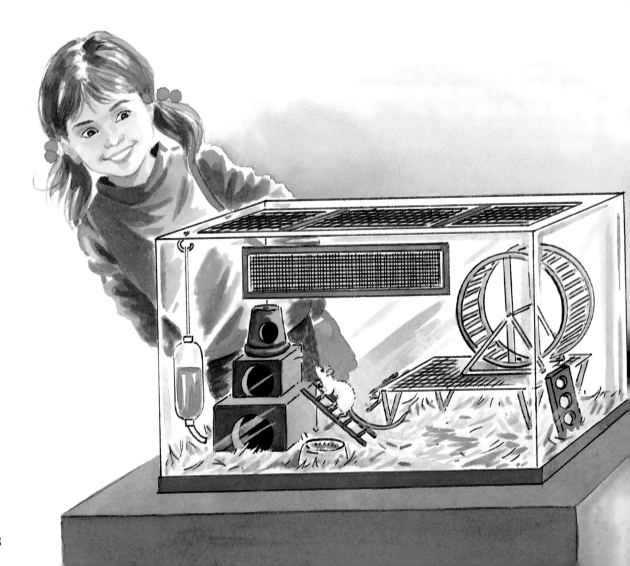

The next day,

a girl came into the shop.

"I have a puppy at home,"

she said.

"If I buy a mouse,

I will have **two** pets."

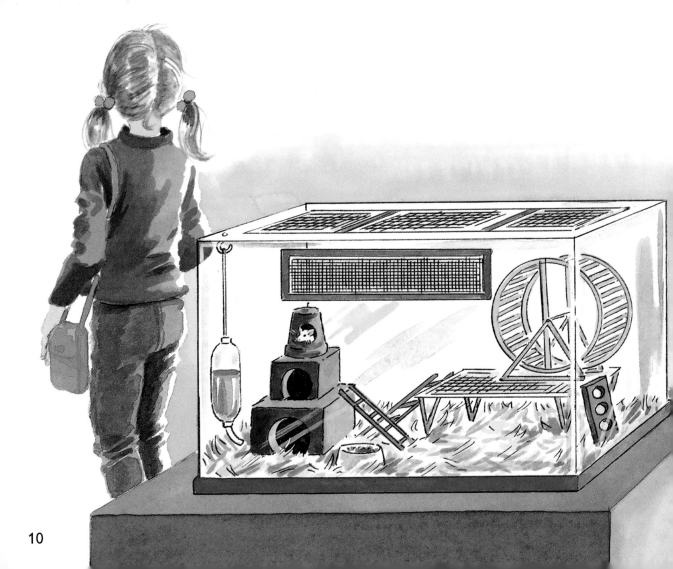

Snowball said, "Puppies eat mice!
I don't want that girl to buy me."

Snowball ran up the ladder
to his little room and hid inside.

The girl walked away.

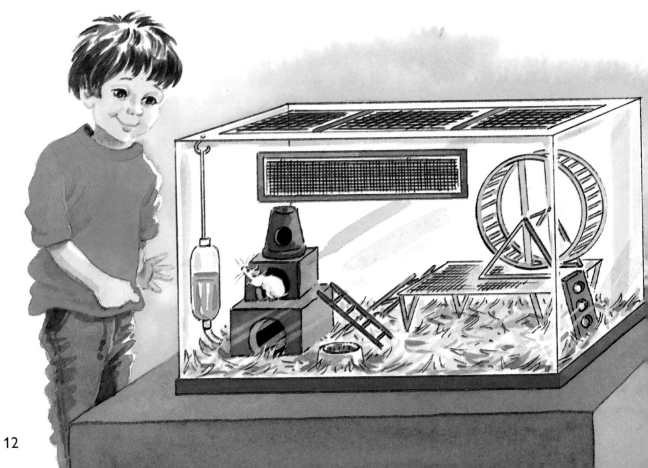

Then a little boy
came into the shop.
"I have a black mouse at home,"
he said.
"If I buy a white mouse,
I will have **two** mice.
They can be friends."

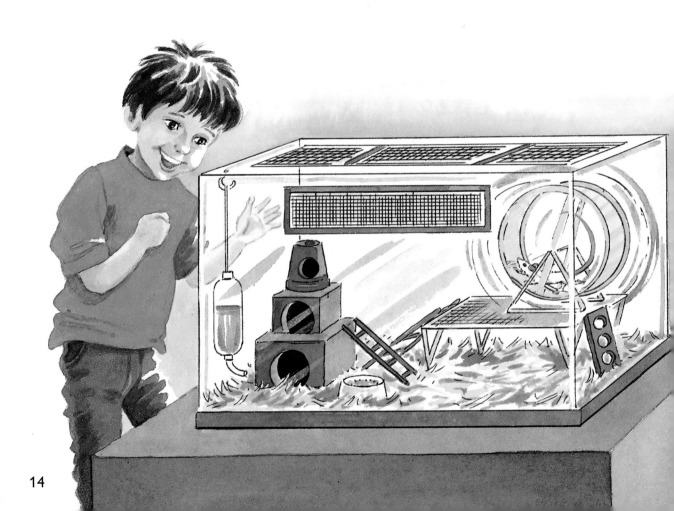

Snowball raced down his ladder.

He jumped inside his wheel.

He ran very fast,

and the wheel went around,

and around, and around.

The little boy smiled at Snowball.

"I will buy you," he said.

So Snowball went home
with the little boy,
and he was very happy.

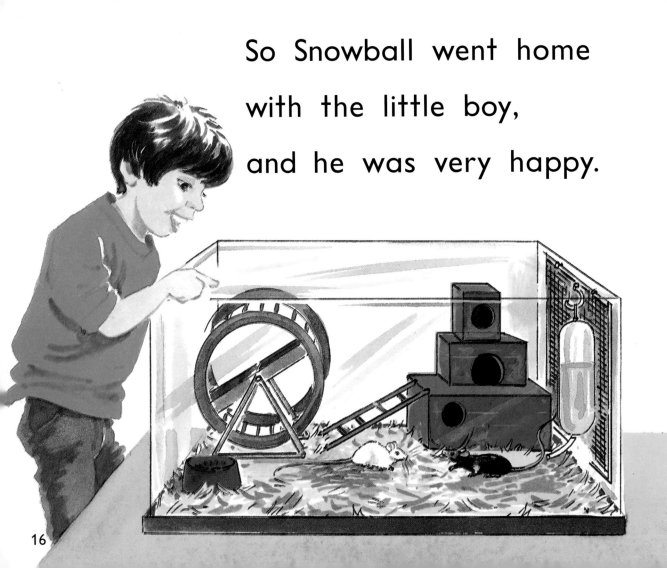